Foods for a Healthy Vagina

Keys to Perfect Vagina Health

Erica Renee Denson

Published in the United States by Kindle Direct Publishing

Foods for a Healthy Vagina: Keys to Perfect Vagina Health

ISBN13- 979-8-874120-29-0

Dedication

I dedicate this book to Jesus Christ my Lord and savior. I prayed for knowledge and he gave me wisdom to navigate the proper things to write.

Thank You

First, I would like to give thanks to Jesus Christ my Lord and savior. Thank you to my dear friend Amos. Amos thank you for shifting my mind to eat healthy and being my biggest supporter. Thank you, Pastor April Gant, for guiding me through the process of book writing.

Table of Contents

Introduction

I'm obsessed with my vagina and her staying healthy. Yes, I talk about my vagina in the third person. Come on ladies y'all know she has a mind of her own sometimes! (Ha Ha!) I have always received compliments about how good my vagina taste and smell. I've never needed to use a plethora of products to maintain a healthy odor-free vagina. I see tons of commercials and products for sale to eliminate odor and cure common vagina issues; however, most vagina issues can be cured and maintained by eating nutritional. Most products that are advertised to cure odors simply mask it. I will give you tips to maintain a healthy vagina daily. Warning: I am not a physician nor am I in the medical

Introduction

field; however, most of my knowledge came from my gynecologist. Although, I did conduct a study with women from different backgrounds and ages to test my theories and products. I've received positive results and feedback from many women; especially, those suffering from menopause and menstrual issues. Most physicians don't want people to use natural healing due to the push of pharmaceutical medications and products.

Chapter 1
Foods

Breakfast

Million-dollar question! What can I eat to maintain a healthy vagina? I will walk you through what a daily meal consists of to maintain a healthy odor-free vagina. Let's start with my love for yogurt.

Yogurt it's a quick satisfying vagina food. Yogurt is a probiotic that has many vagina and digestive health benefits. Yogurt has billions of active cultures such as: Lactobacillus bacteria which is good bacteria for the vagina. Yogurt is packed with many vitamins and minerals to name a few: Zinc, B12, and Magnesium. Yogurt can also help reduce stress. Stress can lead to a disruption in PH balance. PH Balance is your body fluids acidity levels and your natural body alkaline, if your levels

Chapter 1
Foods

become unbalanced the vagina will alert you. Keeping your vagina PH Balance is very important to ward off yeast infections as well as Bacterial Vaginosis (BV). Yogurt will help maintain the proper PH levels. I eat plain or vanilla yogurt to eliminate the extra sugar, which can have a negative effect on your vagina and overall health. If you need flavor in your yogurt spruce it up with fresh fruits. Additionally, yogurt benefits can include better energy levels and a higher sex drive. Good bacteria help to balance acidic levels through the membranes of your vagina secretions. Consume yogurt with active cultures daily to ensure you receive enough good bacteria. If you are not a fan of yogurt, it can be added to a smoothie to disguise the taste, so your vagina will receive all the

Chapter 1
Foods

nutrients it needs to stay healthy. If your PH balance is slightly off, plain yogurt can be inserted into the vagina to help treat and prevent minor irritation caused by yeast infections. Always check with your physician when trying anything new to ensure these foods are safe for your diet.

Flaxseeds are another must-have vagina food. Flaxseeds can be added to yogurt or a smoothie. Flaxseeds are a natural alkaline for your body that will help balance the vagina's PH. Flaxseeds can also help with vagina lubrication. Flaxseeds are overloaded with antioxidants that can balance female hormones. Polyunsaturated fatty acids and protein in Flaxseeds help the vagina's elasticity and promote proper vagina

Chapter 1
Foods

secretions. Some studies have found that Flaxseeds can help remove free radicals from the body that improve stress levels. High-stress levels can cause dryness in the vagina. Many women suffer from vagina dryness due to many factors like menopause and low libido. Flaxseeds can help cure vagina dryness.

Avocado is one of my favorite go-to breakfast vagina foods. I was not always a fan of avocado, but my gynecologist told me it was good for my vagina and I was sold. I tried it and thought, not bad. Avocado is also a natural alkaline fruit as well as filled with monounsaturated fats that can help with vagina lubrication. Avocado can be eaten in many ways: on toast, in a smoothie, and guacamole to name a few. The

Chapter 1
Foods

oil in the avocado help to lubricate the vagina and stimulate cell growth in the lining of the vagina walls.

Watermelon is good for maintaining the proper acidic levels for PH balance. Watermelon has the proper name and it's filled with water which our vagina and body need for hydration. Watermelon is loaded with amino acids and antioxidants, which can improve vagina dryness. Amino acids help build protein that helps with elasticity in the vagina. Watermelon is saturated with many different health benefits that may act as an anti-inflammatory, anticancer effect, and help with muscle soreness. I know this is a book for vagina health, but ladies if your man suffers from Erectile Dysfunction, watermelon rind can

Chapter 1
Foods

help improve blood flow in the male genitals and reward the vagina. Watermelon can be eaten as a snack, juiced, or added to your favorite smoothie.

Lunch

Leafy greens such as kale, spinach, collard greens, and watercress are packed with essential vitamins and minerals that are needed for vagina health. Leafy greens are loaded with water for hydration and help balance your vagina membrane secretions. Leafy greens are naturally acidic vegetables and help naturally balance your PH levels. Make a salad for lunch and give your vagina the nutrients it needs to stimulate lubrication for great orgasms!

Chapter 1
Foods

Cucumber is one of my favorite vegetables for vagina health. Cucumber is made of 96% water, it is naturally alkaline and hydrates the vagina. Any vegetable or fruit that's majority water such as melons and lettuce will hydrate not just your body it will make your vagina well lubricated.

Edamame is a good mid-day snack that will make the vagina very healthy. Edamame is loaded with omega-3 fatty acids and proteins. Proteins in edamame can help generate new cells that maintain the strong lining in the walls of the vagina and help with lubrication. It also contains many minerals and vitamins that can help with menstrual and menopausal symptoms that occur in most women.

Chapter 1
Foods

Nuts are a hand full of protein that is essential for healthy cell growth in the vagina lining. I am a vegetarian "technically" pescatarian because I eat fish occasionally; however, most of my meals are fruits and vegetables an eating habit that can be a challenge to get the proper amount of protein. Nuts and especially almonds provide a natural source of protein, essential to stimulate cell growth in the vagina lining. Almonds have a lot of fatty acids, fiber, and minerals that studies have shown to improve overall vagina health; as well as enhance vagina lubrication.

Almonds are high in zinc, properties that may prevent vagina itching and regulate your menstrual cycle. Almonds can be added to a salad or eaten signally.

Chapter 1
Foods

Dinner

Salmon (wild-caught) is an excellent source of omega-3 fatty acids, protein, and essential vitamins the vagina needs. Fatty acids can provide lubrication to help combat against vagina dryness. Preventing vagina dryness can make intercourse more pleasurable and prevent vagina tears. Protein from fish helps rebuild and maintain cell growth to support the lining of the vagina walls.

Sweet Potatoes are incredibly rich in beta carotene which is converted to vitamin A to support a variety of nutrients the vagina craves.

Chapter 1
Foods

Sweet potatoes are filled with vitamins and minerals that generate healthy cell growth in the vagina as well as stimulate lubrication.

Broccoli has tons of essential nutrients and very high levels of vitamins and minerals. Broccoli is a great source of antioxidants which provides rejuvenation in the vagina. Kaempferol is a natural flavonoid found in broccoli that a study from 2007 found can help defend against ovarian cancer in 40 percent of women.

Cabbage is a low-oxalate leafy green to incorporate into your diet. This water-based green veggie interacts with the mucus membranes in your vagina to make it well-lubricated. Cabbage will Keep those membranes hydrated and help with odor control.

Chapter 1
Foods

Drinks

Kombucha is a probiotic spewing with live cultures that generate good bacteria to fend off harmful bacteria in the vagina. Kombucha is Bursting with millions of active cultures that can help keep the vagina well lubricated. Kombucha is a fermented drink that's very acidic, and if you're like me, I don't drink soda, so Kombucha helps to satisfy my soda cravings. Kombucha is made in a variety of flavors and types. Kombucha helps to regulate and keep away yeast and bacterial infections.

Probiotic Drink is a great alternative to yogurt to build up healthy bacteria. Probiotic drinks are made in different types such as shots, juices, and yogurt blends. Probiotic drinks can be a substitute, for Kombucha if you don't like fermented drinks. As mentioned, probiotics

Chapter 1
Foods

have live bacteria cultures that have been proven to restore and maintain healthy bacteria in the vagina as well as maintain the proper PH balance.

Cranberry Juice, OK ladies, we've all been told to drink cranberry juice; however, the type of juice matters. I was so proud to tell my Gynecologist that I only drink cranberry juice. She asked why? I said for my vagina. She replied cranberry juices are filled with sugar and juice concentrate. She advised me, if I wanted the benefit from cranberries, eat the real thing. I juice cranberries or eat it for a snack. I also put cranberries in my smoothie. Cranberries are tart, so I offset the taste with pineapples or apples blended in my juice or smoothie. Cranberries work wonders for the vagina by producing bacteria that

Chapter 1
Foods

defend against the common Urinary Tract Infections (UTIs) and other bacterial infections.

Lemons are very acidic and can help naturally balance the vagina PH. Lemon juice can be squeezed in your water bottle or make fresh squeezed lemonade. Lemons are loaded with antioxidants that help maintain a healthy vagina.

Chapter 2
Supplements

OK, ladies we've covered most of the nutritional things you can eat to maintain a healthy vagina let's talk about supplements. Vegetarians and vegans have the challenge of ensuring the proper daily consumption of nutrients. It can be difficult to receive enough protein, vitamins, and minerals if you're not consuming enough nutrition daily. Supplements can help fill in the gap if you don't reach the recommended amount from foods. I'll give you an outline of some of the supplements I take daily. Although I consume my leafy greens and fruits sometimes my intake may not fulfill the daily recommended percent of nutrients the vagina and the body need. I want to reiterate that I'm not a doctor nor in the medical field, so anytime you introduce new foods and supplements it's always a

Chapter 2
Supplements

great idea to check with your physician to see if these supplements are healthy for your diet.

Flaxseed supplements are a good source of alpha-linolenic acid to maintain the vagina's PH balance. This supplement is packed with Omega-3 fatty acids that can help build cells in the lining of the vagina walls.

Flax seed supplements also can help with lubrication, especially for women suffering from vagina dryness.

Zinc may help treat vagina dryness, itching, and irritation. Zinc is great for women struggling with menstrual and menopausal issues. Zinc will build a strong vagina lining and help with vagina secretions.

Chapter 2
Supplements

Vitamin A can help stimulate the production of hormones that regulate the vagina as well as keep you energized. Vitamin A help build strong cells in the vagina lining.

Vitamin C help improve blood circulation, which stimulates vagina lubrication.

Chapter 3
Hygiene

Healthy eating is essential for an odor-free lubricated vagina; however, not maintaining proper hygiene will have a negative effect on your overall vagina health. Hygiene and balanced nutrition go hand and hand. I recommend using your hand to wash your vagina. Using your hand to clean your vagina will eliminate the possibility of irritation from laundry detergents and you'll clean it better. I also recommend using a fragrance-free PH balance vagina wash. Fragrance can lead to a yeast infection by causing a disturbance in your PH balance. Fragrance and dyes can also cause vagina dryness and itching. The vagina is not made to smell like perfume it's an open wound and should get air to the area as much as possible. There is a difference between an odor and a

Chapter 3
Hygiene

scent. Every vagina has a scent; however, it should not have an odor. If your vagina has an odor consult with your doctor immediately. The odor from the vagina is a direct indicator that there is a problem. Once you solve any medical issues, these tips can help you maintain a healthy vagina. You should not use fragrance suppositories it could cause vagina irritation, yeast, or UTI infections. Eating healthy and proper hygiene will keep you smelling and tasting fresh and clean.

Chapter 4
Sexual Health

Vagina and Sexual health are one and the same. It is important to maintain both because one can have an adverse effect on the other if precaution is not taken. Ladies, how you care for your vagina will ultimately determine your sexual pleasure as well as orgasms. Everything that enters the vagina should be washed well to prevent yeast and bacterial infections. I wash everything with my vagina soap that enters my vagina including but limited to: fingers, toys, and penis. Fingers should be cleaned with pH-balanced soap with a nail scrubber. Intimate toys can cause vagina bacterial and yeast infections if not cleaned properly. Penis can be washed with vagina soap as well. I make an intimate gesture to clean it, using my hand only, and 99 % of the

Chapter 4
Sexual Health

time it helps get the blood flowing, if you know what I mean, so ladies take the cleaning matter in your hands. (Ha Ha) Men can transmit BV infections. Ladies if you consistently get BV infections from the same partner check with your physician to have them medicated with the same medication you are prescribed or have them see a doctor to prevent the spread back and forth. If you or your partner have multiple sexual partners using protection is the best and only way to prevent and maintain a healthy vagina and keep at bay Sexual Transmitted Diseases (STDs), Sexual Transmitted Infections (STIs), and Bacterial Infections (BV). Sperm is the vagina's worst nightmare as soon as it enters the vagina good bacteria start to attack it due to it being a

Chapter 4
Sexual Health

foreign object. The vagina immediately tries to kill the sperm which disrupts the PH balance. If this is an issue, try to have your partner ejaculate in other areas make it fun and explore, this will help to prevent yeast and BV infections. Oral Sex can disrupt the vagina's PH balance as well. Proper dental hygiene can include, but is not limited to brushing teeth, flossing, and mouthwash before Oral Sex can help prevent yeast and bacterial infections.

Chapter 5
Exercise

Kegel exercises can strengthen your pelvic floor muscles and stimulate better orgasms. Completing 30 to 40 Kegel exercises periodically daily will help build a strong pelvic floor. This type of pelvic exercise will help with bladder control as well as your overall vagina health. The perfect thing about Kegel exercises it can be done discreetly standing, sitting, or laying. Many different exercises target strengthening the pelvic floor such as Squats, Hip Bridges, Hip Roll, Clam Shell, and Reverse Clam Shell. Choose the most comfortable exercise that you can perform to the best of your ability.

Conclusion

This is my vagina bible and tips to maintain a lubricated odor-free vagina. Everybody is different, and certain foods and products have different effects and outcomes; however, proper nutrition and hygiene are unanimous to overall vagina health. Please consult with your physician about everything you read in this book. I am not a doctor! Everyone has different dietary needs and restrictions, so take and apply what you can use that is safe for your health. I hope these tips will give you the positive results it has given many women and me. I make vagina milk that is dairy free, organic, and vegan which will make your vagina super wet-wet. I also make a vagina cleanse that helps maintain a healthy PH balance, especially when there is semen in the vagina. This cleans

Conclusion

can be used daily and immediately after any vagina penetration.

About the Author

Hello readers, my name is Erica Denson. I'm a mother and Grandmother. Eating healthy is a passion for me and provides many health benefits. I always found myself giving woman advise about health, due to my own personal experiences. Consistently hearing from women that they battle with bacterial and yeast infection became a concern. Working closely with my gynecologist and researching my diet, lead me to study different women and how I could help change the narrative. From the study, I learned what helped women maintain a healthy vagina. Eat to live not live to eat!

CTA

Please contact me, for purchase information, samples, and any questions: healthyv@vaginahealthy.org